MW01232045

SOMATIC EXERCISES FOR WEIGHT LOSS

30 DAILY ROUTINES AND EXERCISES TO
INCREASE FLEXIBILITY, STRENGTH, AND
BALANCE FOR PHYSICAL AND EMOTIONAL
WELL-BEING

OLIVIA WELLNESS

1

HOW TO USE THIS BOOK

Welcome to "Somatic Exercises for Weight Loss"! As the author of this book, I'm thrilled to guide you through a transformative journey toward better health and wellness. Let me walk you through what you'll find in each section of the book so you can make the most out of it:

1. Understanding and Benefits of Somatic Exercises for Weight Loss

Here, I lay the groundwork for somatic exercises and how they can significantly aid your weight loss and overall health journey. You'll also find inspiring success stories to motivate you on your path.

2. *Warm-Up and Stretching*

This section is your starting point for each exercise session. I've compiled a variety of warm-up exercises and stretching routines to prepare your body, improve your flexibility, and prevent injuries. You'll learn both dynamic and static stretching techniques.

3. Basic Exercises

This section is for you if you're new to somatic exercises or prefer gentler movements. It focuses on building your body awareness and engaging in fluid, mindful movements, making it perfect for beginners.

4. Intermediate Exercises

Ready to step up your game? This section introduces exercises that are more challenging and ideal for those comfortable with the basics and eager to progress further.

5. Advanced Exercises

For those looking for a deeper level of challenge, the advanced exercises in this section will test your body awareness and control, offering an intense and rewarding experience.

6. Daily Routines

In this part, I've put together daily routines that blend exercises from various levels. These routines are designed to provide well-rounded workouts to suit different fitness goals and levels.

7. Nutritional Advice

A vital part of any weight loss journey is nutrition. This section offers fundamental nutritional advice to complement your exercise routine, focusing on balanced eating habits and healthy food choices.

8. Conclusion

As we wrap up, I'll revisit the key points from the book and offer some final words of encouragement. Remember, your journey to wellness is ongoing, and consistency is key.

9. *Appendix*

Finally, the appendix contains a glossary of terms, additional resources, and references for those who want to explore further.

You should approach this book as a journey rather than a destination. Start where you feel comfortable, and gradually build your practice. Remember, this book is a guide and a companion on your path to a healthier, more balanced life. Enjoy the journey!

Customizing Your Routine

As you embark on this journey with "Somatic Exercises for Weight Loss," you must recognize that each individual's path to wellness is unique. Customizing that's your routine to fit your specific fitness levels and goals is crucial. Let me guide you through how to tailor these exercises and routines to make them your own.

Start by taking a moment to assess your current fitness level. It's essential to be honest and realistic in this self-assessment. Whether you're a beginner, intermediate, or advanced in physical activity, this understanding will help you pick the right point to start in this book.

Next, think about your goals. Are you aiming for weight loss, better flexibility, reduced stress, or overall health improvement? Your objectives will steer the direction of your routine customization. This clarity in your goals will be your compass as you navigate the exercises. If you're new to somatic exercises, I recommend easing into them with the basic exercises, no matter how simple they seem. These foundational exercises are pivotal in building your body awareness and mindfulness – crucial elements in somatic practice.

Listening to your body is at the heart of bodily exercises. As you progress through the routines, pay close attention to how your body feels during and after each exercise. This internal dialogue with your body will guide you in adjusting the intensity and choice of exercises. It's a signal to modify your approach if something feels overly challenging or uncomfortable. Feel empowered to mix and match exercises from different sections of the book. As you grow stronger and more in tune with your body, blending basic with intermediate or advanced exercises can keep your routine dynamic and challenging.

Consistency in your routine will be a key factor in your success. Establishing a routine that aligns with your daily life and sticking to it is more beneficial than occasional intense workouts. This could mean shorter or longer daily sessions a few times a week. Find a rhythm that harmonizes with your lifestyle. As you get stronger and more confident in the exercises, challenge yourself. This could mean progressing to more advanced exercises, increasing the duration of your sessions, or exploring more demanding routines. Your routine should evolve as you do.

Remember, nutrition is an integral part of your journey. The nutritional advice in this book isn't just a supplement to your exercise routine; it's a cornerstone of your overall wellness plan. Embracing healthy eating habits will augment the benefits of your somatic exercises.

Documenting your progress can serve as a powerful motivational tool. Keeping a journal where you note down your exercises, feelings, and changes in your body and mind can help you track your journey and celebrate your achievements, no matter how small they seem. Lastly, be patient and kind to yourself. This journey is about self-improvement, not instant results. Every small step you take is an achievement worth celebrating. Embrace this journey with self-compassion, and let each day bring you closer to your wellness goals. By following these principles, you'll be able to craft a somatic exercise routine that's not only effective but also deeply personal. This book is here to guide you, but the journey is yours to shape. Let's begin this path to wellness together with a routine that's as unique as you are.

Consistency and Progress Tracking

In your journey through "Somatic Exercises for Weight Loss," one of the critical elements to success is consistency in your practice. Regular exercise, mindfulness, and a deep connection to your body's needs can lead to profound and lasting changes. But how do you ensure consistency and effectively track your progress? Let's delve into this. Consistency is more than just exercising regularly; it's about making your practice a seamless part of your daily routine. It's about finding joy and value in each movement and mindfulness moment. Set realistic goals and a schedule that fits your lifestyle to cultivate this habit. Whether it's a few minutes each morning or a longer session several times a week, what matters most is that it's manage-able and enjoyable for you.

But how do you know if you're making progress? This is where tracking comes into play. Keep an exercise diary. Depending on your preference, this diary can be a simple notebook, a digital document, or even a specialized app. The key is to use it to reflect on your journey, track your routines, and observe your body and mind changes. In your diary, note your exercises, their duration, and how you felt before and after each session. This will not only help you keep track of what you've done but also allow you to tune into your body's responses to different exercises. Over time, you might notice patterns emerging – certain exercises that make you feel particularly good or some that you find challenging. Also, use your diary to record other important aspects of your wellness journey, like changes in your sleeping patterns, stress levels, and eating habits. All these elements are interconnected, and observing them can give you a holistic view of your progress.

Remember, progress in somatic exercises isn't just about physical changes. It's about how you feel in your body, the level of stress you experience, and your overall sense of well-being. So, in your diary, make space for personal reflections. How are you feeling mentally and emotionally? Are you noticing changes in your stress levels or mood? These observations are just as important as the physical ones. From time to time, look back through your diary. You'll be able to see just how far you've come, which is incredibly motivating. It's a tangible record of your commitment to yourself and your health. And on days when motivation is low, it serves as a powerful reminder of why you started this journey and the progress you've made. Consistency in practice and tracking your progress are your allies in this journey. They provide structure, motivation, and a clear path to seeing the changes you're working towards. Let's use these tools to build a routine that not only brings you closer to your fitness goals but also enhances your overall well-being.

Safety Tips and Precautions

When embarking on any new exercise regimen, particularly one involving somatic exercises, it's crucial to prioritize safety to avoid injury and ensure a positive experience, especially for beginners or those with specific health concerns. In this section of "Somatic Exercises for Weight Loss," I'd like to share some essential safety tips and precautions.

Start Slowly and Gently: If you're new to somatic exercises or returning to physical activity after a break, it's essential to start slowly. Allow your body to get used to the new movements gradually. You are rushing into the risk of injury. Begin with basic exercises and slowly increase the intensity as your body becomes more accustomed to the movements.

Warm-Up and Cool Down: A proper warm-up before starting your exercise routine is crucial. It prepares your muscles and joints for the workout, reducing the risk of strains or injuries. Similarly, cooling down after your exercises helps your body to return to its resting state slowly and can prevent muscle stiffness.

Listen to Your Body: Somatic exercises are all about being in tune with your body. Pay close attention to how your body feels during the exercises. If you experience pain or discomfort, stop immediately. It's essential to differentiate between the natural effort of exercise and pain that could signal an injury.

Maintain Proper Form: Ensure that you are performing each exercise with the correct form. This is not only vital for the effectiveness of the exercise but also for preventing injuries. If you need clarification on the correct form, consider seeking guidance from a qualified instructor.

Stay Hydrated and Nourished: Drink plenty of water before, during, and after your exercise sessions. Proper hydration is crucial for physical performance and recovery. Also, ensure you're eating a balanced diet to fuel your body with the necessary nutrients.

Consult with Healthcare Professionals: If you have any existing health concerns, injuries, or conditions, consult with a healthcare professional before starting a new exercise routine. They can provide advice tailored to your specific needs and help you identify any exercises you should avoid.

Avoid Overexertion: While it's good to challenge yourself, overexertion can lead to injuries. Be aware of your current fitness level, and don't push your body beyond its limits. Remember, somatic exercises are about mindful movements, not about pushing through pain or fatigue.

Use Proper Equipment and Environment: If any exercise requires equipment, make sure it is in good condition and suitable for the activity. Also, ensure that your exercise environment is safe – the floor should be non-slip, and there should be enough space to move around freely.

Regular Rest and Recovery: Allow your body time to rest and recover, especially after intense sessions. Regular rest days are essential for muscle recovery and overall physical health.

By following these safety tips and precautions, you can enjoy the full benefits of somatic exercises while minimizing the risk of injury. Remember, the goal of these exercises is to enhance your overall well-being, and that includes taking care of your body by practicing safely and responsibly.

Encouragement for Persistence and Patience

Embarking on a fitness journey, especially one involving somatic exercises for weight loss and overall well-being, is a commendable endeavor. However, it's crucial to acknowledge that real, lasting change takes time and dedication. In this part of the book, I want to offer you a motivational note on the importance of persistence and patience in your journey. First and foremost, understand that progress is not always linear. There will be days when you feel like you've taken two steps forward and one step back. This is completely normal and part of the process. The key is not to get discouraged by these moments but to see them as opportunities for learning and growth. Remember, every small step you take is a victory. Whether it's completing a workout, feeling a little more flexible, or simply being more mindful of your body throughout the day, these are all signs of progress. Celebrate these small wins; they add up over time and contribute significantly to your overall success. It's also important to listen to your body and respect its limits. Somatic exercises are about creating harmony between your mind and body, not pushing through pain or discomfort. If your body is telling you to slow down or take a break, listen to it. Rest and recovery are just as important as the exercises themselves. Be patient with yourself. Changes in your body, whether it's weight loss, increased flexibility, or improved muscle tone, will happen gradually. Trust in the process and the exercises you're doing. Your body is an incredible machine, and with consistent effort, it will respond positively.

Stay persistent. There will be days when motivation is low, and that's okay. What's important is to keep going, even if it's just a few minutes of exercise a day. Consistency is key. Over time, these exercises will become a natural part of your routine, something you look forward to rather than a chore. Lastly, remember why you started this journey. Keep your goals in mind, whether they're related to weight loss, health, stress reduction, or simply wanting to feel better in your body. Your reasons for starting are your anchor, keeping you grounded and focused when challenges arise.

Be kind to yourself, celebrate your progress, no matter how small, and stay the course. The path to wellness is a journey, not a destination, and it's worth every step. With persistence, patience, and a positive mindset, you're capable of achieving incredible things. Let's continue this journey together, with the understanding that every step forward is a step toward a healthier, happier you.

2

UNDERSTANDING AND BENEFITS OF SOMATIC EXERCISES FOR WEIGHT LOSS

Definition of Somatic Exercises

Somatic exercises, at their core, are a form of movement therapy that emphasizes internal physical perception and experience. Unlike traditional exercises that often focus on external appearance and objective performance metrics, somatic exercises are about tuning into the body's internal sensations and responses. The term "somatic" is derived from the Greek word "soma," which means "living body." This approach to exercise is rooted in the understanding that mind and body are not separate entities but are deeply interconnected. By focusing on the internal experience of movement, somatic exercises aim to improve the communication between the mind and the body.

These exercises typically involve slow, gentle movements that are less about exerting effort and more about developing a deeper awareness of the body's capabilities and limitations. The goal is to move in ways that feel good and natural rather than pushing the body to its limits.

Emphasis on Internal Perception and Experience

The uniqueness of somatic exercises lies in their emphasis on internal perception and experience. Practitioners are encouraged to pay close attention to how their bodies feel during each movement, noting any sensations of tension, relaxation, discomfort, or ease. This mindfulness approach helps individuals develop a heightened sense of body awareness, which is crucial for overall well-being. In somatic exercises, the quality of movement is valued over quantity. The idea is to perform each movement with intention and focus, creating a harmonious dialogue between the body and the mind. This approach helps individuals become more attuned to their body's needs and responses, leading to a more intuitive and self-aware form of physical activity.

Benefits for Weight Loss

Somatic exercises are particularly beneficial for weight loss for several reasons:

- *Stress Reduction:* By focusing on the mind-body connection, these exercises help reduce stress, which is a significant factor in weight gain and difficulty in losing weight.

- *Improved Metabolism:* As individuals become more in tune with their bodies, they often make healthier lifestyle choices, leading to improved metabolism.

- *Enhanced Digestive Function:* The gentle movements and deep breathing associated with somatic exercises can improve digestion and aid in more efficient nutrient absorption and waste elimination.

- *Fat Burning:* While not as intense as traditional aerobic exercises, somatic exercises still help burn calories and increase muscle tone, contributing to fat loss over time.

- *Sustainable Practice:* Since somatic exercises are gentle and enjoyable, individuals are more likely to stick with them long-term, making them a sustainable part of a weight loss journey.

Somatic exercises offer a unique approach to weight loss that goes beyond traditional exercise methods. By focusing on the internal experience of movement, they foster a deeper connection between mind and body, leading to holistic health improvements and sustainable weight management.

Connection Between Mind and Body

The connection between mind and body is a foundational aspect of somatic exercises, playing a crucial role in their effectiveness and appeal. Somatic exercises enhance this mind-body connection, leading to more mindful and effective workouts. This section explores how these exercises bridge the gap between mental and physical health, contributing to a more holistic approach to fitness and well-being.

- *Enhanced Mindfulness:* Somatic exercises require practitioners to be fully present in the moment, focusing intensely on the sensations and movements of their bodies. This heightened state of mindfulness during exercise ensures that each movement is performed with intention and awareness, fostering a greater connection between mental and physical states.

- *Improved Body Awareness:* By concentrating on internal sensations and responses, individuals practicing somatic exercises develop a keener awareness of their bodies. This awareness is not just about recognizing discomfort or tension but also about understanding the body's capabilities, strengths, and limitations. It encourages a more nuanced and respectful approach to exercise and body care.

- *Emotional Regulation:* The mind-body connection highlighted in somatic exercises also plays a role in emotional regulation. Physical movement can be a powerful tool for expressing and processing emotions. Somatic exercises, with their focus on internal experience, allow individuals to explore and release emotional tensions, leading to improved mental health and emotional well-being.

- *Stress Reduction and Relaxation:* By promoting a calm and focused state of mind, somatic exercises are effective in reducing stress and anxiety. The practice encourages a relaxation response in the body, which is beneficial not only for mental health but also for physical health, as it can reduce the risk of stress-related disorders.

- *Cognitive Benefits:* Engaging in somatic exercises has been shown to have cognitive benefits. The focus and concentration required during these exercises can enhance mental clarity, improve attention span, and even boost creativity. This cognitive engagement makes workouts not just physically beneficial but also mentally stimulating.

The connection between mind and body is a crucial element that makes somatic exercises especially effective. This approach not only enhances physical fitness but also contributes to mental and emotional well-being, making it a comprehensive method for overall health improvement. The integration of psychological and physical aspects in exercise routines leads to a more balanced, mindful, and fulfilling workout experience.

Benefits for Weight Loss

Somatic exercises contribute significantly to weight loss and overall health improvement through a variety of mechanisms. These exercises offer a holistic approach, impacting not just the physical body but also mental and emotional well-being, which are key factors in weight management. Here's a detailed look at how somatic exercises facilitate weight loss:

- *Improved Metabolism:* Regular practice of somatic exercises can lead to an improved metabolic rate. The gentle yet engaging nature of these exercises helps in building lean muscle mass, which in turn increases the body's resting metabolic rate. A higher metabolic rate means the body burns more calories even when at rest, aiding in weight loss and management.

- *Better Digestion:* The movements in somatic exercises often involve the core and abdominal muscles, which can positively affect the digestive system. Improved digestion means the body is more efficient at processing food and eliminating waste, reducing issues like bloating and constipation. This efficiency is crucial for weight loss as it ensures that the body is absorbing nutrients effectively and maintaining a healthy gut.

- *Reduced Stress Levels:* Stress has a direct link to weight gain, particularly in the form of visceral fat around the abdomen. Somatic exercises, with their focus on mindfulness and body awareness, can significantly reduce stress levels. Lower stress levels lead to a decrease in cortisol, a hormone associated with fat accumulation, thereby aiding in weight loss.

- *More Efficient Fat Burning:* While somatic exercises may not be as high-intensity as some other forms of exercise, they still play a role in burning fat. By improving overall muscle tone and increasing body awareness, these exercises help individuals engage in more efficient and effective workouts. Additionally, the relaxation and stress-reducing aspects of somatic exercises can shift the body from a fat-storage mode to a fat-burning mode.

- *Holistic Health Improvement:* Somatic exercises encourage an overall healthier lifestyle. As individuals become more attuned to their bodies, they are more likely to make healthier food choices and adopt other habits conducive to weight loss and maintenance. This holistic approach is often more sustainable and effective in the long term compared to drastic diets or intense workout regimens.

Somatic exercises offer a comprehensive approach to weight loss. They not only provide physical benefits like improved metabolism and digestion but also contribute to mental and emotional well-being, which is crucial for sustainable weight management. By integrating these exercises into a regular fitness routine, individuals can enjoy a more balanced, healthy lifestyle that supports their weight loss goals.

Long-term Health Benefits

Somatic exercises offer a range of long-term health and wellness benefits, making them an invaluable part of a sustained healthy lifestyle. These exercises go beyond immediate physical fitness, contributing to lasting improvements in various aspects of health. Here are some of the critical long-term benefits:

- *Increased Flexibility:* Regular practice of somatic exercises helps in gradually increasing the body's flexibility. This is achieved through gentle stretching and mindful movements that encourage the muscles and joints to loosen and lengthen. Increased flexibility reduces the risk of injuries and improves overall mobility, making daily activities more accessible and more comfortable.

- *Stronger Muscles:* While somatic exercises are not typically high-impact or high-intensity, they are very effective in strengthening the muscles, especially the deep core muscles that are often overlooked in conventional workouts. This muscle strengthening is more about stability and endurance than bulk, leading to a stronger, more toned body that functions efficiently in both daily activities and more strenuous physical tasks.

- *Improved Posture:* Somatic exercises emphasize body alignment and balance, which naturally lead to improved posture. By strengthening the core and enhancing body awareness, these exercises help individuals maintain a natural, comfortable posture, reducing the strain on the spine and joints. Good posture is not only important for appearance but also for preventing back pain and other musculoskeletal issues.

- *Enhanced Overall Well-being:* The holistic nature of somatic exercises means they offer benefits that extend beyond physical health. These exercises have been shown to reduce stress, improve mental clarity, and enhance emotional balance. The focus on mindful movement and body awareness helps in developing a deeper connection with oneself, contributing to an overall sense of well-being.

- *Prevention of Chronic Conditions:* Regular engagement in somatic exercises can play a role in preventing various chronic conditions such as arthritis, osteoporosis, and heart disease. The gentle yet effective movements improve circulation, bone density, and heart health, making these exercises particularly beneficial for aging populations.

- *Sustainable Fitness Routine:* One of the most significant benefits of somatic exercises is their sustainability. Because they are gentle and adaptable, they can be practiced by individuals of all ages and fitness levels and can easily be incorporated into a daily routine. This accessibility ensures that the benefits of the exercises are not just temporary but can be maintained over a lifetime.

The long-term health and wellness benefits of somatic exercises are extensive. They offer a comprehensive approach to health, addressing physical, mental, and emotional aspects. By incorporating somatic exercises into their routines, individuals can enjoy increased flexibility, stronger muscles, improved posture, and an overall enhancement in their quality of life.

Practical Exercises

As you embark on the practical exercise section of this book, I'm excited to share with you the very same routines and poses that I offer to my private clients. These exercises have been carefully selected and structured to ensure that you can perform them independently and effectively, just by reading the descriptions. My aim is to provide you with clear, easy-to-understand instructions that empower you to carry out each movement with confidence and autonomy. Each pose and routine described in this book is crafted to be self-explanatory, eliminating the need for visual aids. The detailed descriptions are designed to guide you through each exercise, helping you visualize and execute the movements accurately. This approach fosters a deeper understanding and connection with your body, enhancing the effectiveness of each exercise.

While I strive to make each instruction as clear as possible, I understand that sometimes seeing a movement in action can provide additional clarity. If you find yourself needing a visual reference for any of the exercises, a simple search on a video platform like YouTube, using the name of the pose, can offer you supplementary guidance. This way, you can ensure you're performing each movement correctly and safely.

I have arranged a unique and user-friendly layout to enhance your learning and practice experience. Each left-hand page details a specific exercise, complete with its practical explanation. This approach is designed to guide you step-by-step through the execution of each movement, ensuring you can perform the exercise correctly and effectively.

On the right-hand page corresponding to each exercise, you'll find valuable tips and notes. These insights are aimed at enriching your understanding of the exercise, providing additional context, and offering guidance to refine your technique. This could include modifications for different fitness levels, common mistakes to avoid, benefits of the exercise, and how it contributes to your overall wellness journey.

This dual-page layout has been thoughtfully designed to provide a comprehensive learning experience. It ensures that you have all the necessary information at your fingertips, facilitating a deeper engagement with each exercise. Whether you are a beginner or more advanced in your fitness journey, these additional insights will help you tailor the exercises to your individual needs and goals.

Remember, the journey to wellness is personal and ever-evolving. These exercises, along with the accompanying tips and notes, are here to support you on your path to improved health and well-being.

Levels of experience and fitness (you can combine them in the future)

- **Warm-Up and Stretching**

These exercises are designed to prepare your body for the workout ahead. They include both dynamic and static stretching routines, perfect for getting your muscles ready and preventing injuries.

- **Basic Exercises**

Ideal for beginners or those looking to focus on body awareness and fluid movement, these exercises form the foundation of a good fitness routine.

- **Intermediate Exercises**

As you progress, these exercises will help you step up in terms of intensity and complexity, offering a balanced challenge for your developing skills.

- **Advanced Exercises**

For those who are ready for a more challenging routine, these exercises demand a good level of body awareness and offer a higher degree of difficulty.

Remember, this journey is about your personal growth and well-being. Each exercise is a step towards a healthier, more balanced you. Whether you're a beginner or an experienced fitness enthusiast, there's something in here for everyone.

WARM-UP EXERCISES TO PREPARE THE BODY

Jogging on the Spot

How to Perform Jogging on the Spot

1. Starting Position: Stand upright with your feet hip-width apart. Keep your back straight, shoulders relaxed, and look forward.

2. Arm Movement: Bend your arms at the elbows. As you jog, swing your arms back and forth in rhythm with your legs. Keep your hands relaxed.

3. Leg Movement: Begin to lift your feet off the ground in a light jogging motion. Your knees should lift slightly with each step.

4. Pace: Start with a slow pace to gradually warm up your body. As you feel more comfortable, you can increase the speed to raise your heart rate further.

5. Breathing: Maintain steady, even breaths. Inhale and exhale rhythmically to ensure a steady supply of oxygen during the exercise.

6. Duration: Continue jogging on the spot for about 3-5 minutes, depending on your fitness level.

Jogging on the Spot

Tips

- Keep your movements light and bouncy. Avoid heavy stomping to reduce impact on your joints.
- Focus on engaging your core muscles to maintain balance and stability.
- Keep your gaze forward and your head up to maintain a neutral neck position.

Note

Jogging on the spot is an excellent warm-up exercise as it gently increases your heart rate and warms up your muscles, preparing your body for more intensive workouts.

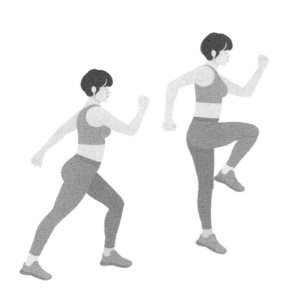

If you find yourself needing a visual reference for any of the exercises, a simple search on a video platform like YouTube, using the name of the pose, can offer you supplementary guidance. This way, you can ensure you're performing each movement correctly and safely.

Hip Circles

How to Perform Hip Circles

1. Starting Position: Stand with your feet shoulder-width apart. Keep your knees slightly bent for stability.
2. Hand Position: Place your hands on your hips or rest them on your waist.
3. The Movement: Gently push your hips forward, then to the side, backward, and to the other side, creating a circular motion. Imagine drawing a circle with your hips.
4. Range of Motion: Start with smaller circles, and as your hips begin to loosen, gradually increase the size of the circles.
5. Direction: After completing several circles in one direction, switch and rotate your hips in the opposite direction.
6. Rhythm and Breathing: Maintain a slow and controlled pace, coordinating your breath with the movement. Inhale as you move your hips forward and exhale as you move them backward.
7. Duration: Continue performing hip circles for about 1-2 minutes, or until you feel your hip area is adequately warmed up.

Hip Circles

Tips

- Keep your upper body as still as possible, focusing the movement in the hips.
- Avoid rushing the circles. The effectiveness of this exercise lies in its slow, deliberate motion.
- Pay attention to any tightness or restrictions in your hip movement and work within your comfortable range of motion.

Note

Hip circles are excellent for enhancing hip mobility, which is essential for overall lower body flexibility and function.

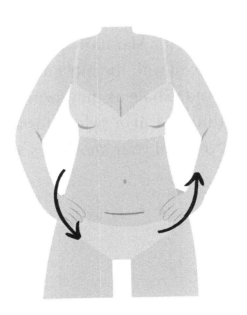

If you find yourself needing a visual reference for any of the exercises, a simple search on a video platform like YouTube, using the name of the pose, can offer you supplementary guidance. This way, you can ensure you're performing each movement correctly and safely.

Arm Swings

How to Perform Arm Swings

1. Starting Position: Stand with your feet shoulder-width apart. Keep your knees slightly bent and your back straight.
2. Arm Position: Extend your arms out to the sides at shoulder height.
3. The Movement: Begin to swing your arms gently in front of your body and then behind, in a steady and controlled motion. The arms should cross in front of your chest when swinging forward.
4. Range of Motion: Gradually increase the range of motion as your muscles warm up. Ensure that the movement is coming from your shoulders.
5. Rhythm and Breathing: Maintain a rhythmic pace and coordinate your breath with the movement – inhale as your arms swing back and exhale as they swing forward.
6. Duration: Continue the arm swings for about 30-60 seconds, or until you feel your shoulders and chest have warmed up.

Arm Swings

Tips

- Keep your movements fluid and avoid jerky motions to prevent strain.
- Focus on relaxing your shoulders as you swing your arms. Avoid tensing up your neck or upper back.
- As you progress, you can increase the speed of your swings slightly, but always prioritize control and range of motion over speed.

Note

Arm swings are an effective way to warm up the shoulders and chest, preparing them for more strenuous activities.

This is another method to practice this exercise

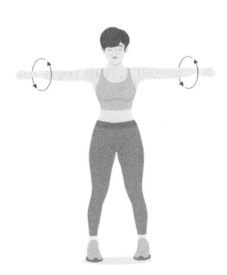

If you find yourself needing a visual reference for any of the exercises, a simple search on a video platform like YouTube, using the name of the pose, can offer you supplementary guidance. This way, you can ensure you're performing each movement correctly and safely.

Spinal Twists

How to Perform Spinal Twists

1. Starting Position: Sit on the floor with your legs extended in front of you. Keep your back straight and your shoulders relaxed.
2. Leg Position: Bend your right knee and place your right foot on the outside of your left knee. Keep your left leg straight or you can bend it with your left foot near your right buttock, if comfortable.
3. Twist Movement: Turn your upper body to the right. Place your left elbow on the outside of your right knee and your right hand on the floor behind you for support.
4. Gaze and Upper Body: As you twist, turn your head to look over your right shoulder if it's comfortable for your neck. Ensure that the twist is initiated from your lower back, moving up to the upper back, and then the neck.
5. Breathing: Inhale deeply as you sit up tall, and exhale as you deepen the twist. Keep your breathing steady and deep.
6. Hold and Switch Sides: Hold the twist for about 20-30 seconds, then release and repeat on the other side.

Spinal Twists

Tips

- It's important to keep your spine straight and elongated during the twist. Avoid slouching or rounding your back.
- Move into the twist gently and slowly. Do not force your body into a deeper twist than is comfortable.
- Focus on the sensation of the twist rather than how far you can turn. The aim is to increase spinal mobility, not to push into discomfort.
- If you experience any pain, especially in the lower back or neck, ease off the twist and consult with a healthcare professional if necessary.

Note

Spinal twists are excellent for increasing spinal mobility, improving digestion, and relieving tension in the back. They help to stretch the back muscles and spine, promoting flexibility and relaxation.

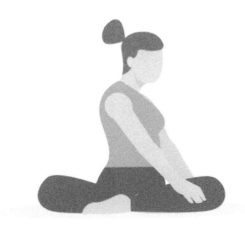

If you find yourself needing a visual reference for any of the exercises, a simple search on a video platform like YouTube, using the name of the pose, can offer you supplementary guidance. This way, you can ensure you're performing each movement correctly and safely.

Knee Lifts

How to Perform Knee Lifts

1. Starting Position: Stand tall with your feet hip-width apart. Keep your back straight, and your arms at your sides or place your hands on your hips for balance.
2. The Movement: Slowly lift one knee towards your chest while keeping the other leg straight and stable. Raise the knee as high as comfortably possible without straining.
3. Balance: Focus on maintaining your balance. If needed, hold onto a chair or wall for support.
4. Alternate Legs: Lower the lifted knee back to the starting position and then lift the other knee. Alternate between legs with a smooth and controlled motion.
5. Breathing: Inhale as you lift your knee and exhale as you lower it back down.
6. Duration: Perform this exercise for about 1-2 minutes, alternating knees.

Knee Lifts

Tips

- Keep your movements controlled. Avoid jerky or rushed motions to prevent any strain on your joints.
- Engage your core muscles throughout the exercise to help with balance and stability.
- Keep your lifted foot flexed to engage the muscles in your leg more effectively.
- As you progress, try to lift your knee higher to increase the range of motion and intensity of the exercise.

Note

Knee lifts are a great way to activate your leg muscles and glutes, and they also help improve balance and coordination.

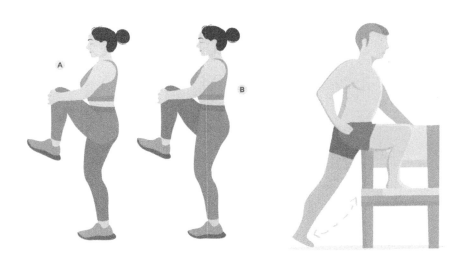

If you find yourself needing a visual reference for any of the exercises, a simple search on a video platform like YouTube, using the name of the pose, can offer you supplementary guidance. This way, you can ensure you're performing each movement correctly and safely.

DYNAMIC AND STATIC STRETCHING

Arm and Shoulder Stretch

How to Perform Arm and Shoulder Stretch

1. Starting Position: Stand with your feet shoulder-width apart. Keep your knees slightly bent and your body relaxed.
2. Arm Swings: Extend your arms out to your sides at shoulder height. Swing them slowly in front of your chest and then open them back out wide. Continue this movement in a controlled manner for about 30 seconds.
3. Shoulder Circles: Next, perform shoulder circles. Lift your shoulders up towards your ears, then roll them backward, down, and then forward in a circular motion. Do this for about 20 seconds, then reverse the direction for another 20 seconds.
4. Cross-Body Arm Stretch: Extend one arm straight across your chest. Use your other hand to gently pull the extended arm closer to your chest, stretching the shoulder. Hold for about 15 seconds, then switch arms.
5. Tricep Stretch: Lift one arm overhead, then bend your elbow so that your hand reaches towards the opposite shoulder blade. Use your other hand to gently press on the bent elbow for a deeper stretch. Hold for 15 seconds, then switch arms.
6. Rhythm and Breathing: Keep your movements smooth and coordinated with your breathing. Inhale during the initial phase of the stretch and exhale as you deepen the stretch.

Arm and Shoulder Stretch

Tips

- Ensure that your movements are fluid and controlled. Avoid jerking or bouncing, as this can cause muscle strain.
- For the cross-body and tricep stretches, be careful not to pull or push too hard. The stretch should feel comfortable and not painful.
- Keep your neck relaxed and your posture upright during the stretches. Avoid slumping or leaning to one side.
- If you feel any pain, especially in the shoulder joints, stop immediately and consult a healthcare professional.

Note

Arm and shoulder stretches are essential for maintaining flexibility and range of motion in the upper body. They are particularly beneficial for individuals who spend a lot of time at a desk or in front of a computer, as they help relieve tension and prevent stiffness in the arms, shoulders, and upper back. These dynamic stretches warm up the muscles, making them an excellent preparation for upper-body intensive activities.

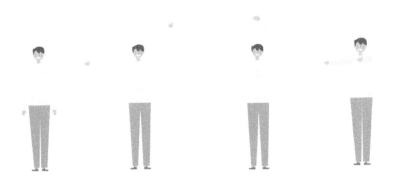

If you find yourself needing a visual reference for any of the exercises, a simple search on a video platform like YouTube, using the name of the pose, can offer you supplementary guidance. This way, you can ensure you're performing each movement correctly and safely.

Standing Toe Touches

How to Perform Standing Toe Touches

1. Starting Position: Stand with your feet hip-width apart. Keep your knees slightly bent to avoid strain on your lower back.

2. The Movement: Inhale and slowly extend your arms above your head. As you exhale, hinge at your hips and bend forward, reaching towards your toes. Keep your back straight as you lower down.

3. Touch and Return: Try to touch your toes, but if you can't reach them, go as far as comfortable, whether that's your shins or knees. Hold the position for a few seconds.

4. Rising Up: Inhale as you slowly roll back up to the standing position, vertebra by vertebra, keeping your back straight. Your head should come up last.

5. Repetition: Repeat this stretch 5-10 times, each time trying to stretch a little further, but always within your comfort zone.

Standing Toe Touches

Tips

- Focus on keeping the movement fluid and controlled. Avoid any jerky motions which can lead to muscle strain.
- It's important to keep the knees slightly bent, especially if you have tight hamstrings or lower back issues.
- This stretch targets the hamstrings and lower back, so you should feel a gentle pull in these areas, but no pain.
- Ensure that the bend is coming from your hips, not your waist, to maximize the stretch in the back of your legs.
- Breathe deeply throughout the stretch, as this will help deepen the stretch and relax your muscles.

Note

Standing toe touches are an excellent dynamic stretch for the back of the legs and the lower back. They help to improve flexibility in the hamstrings and can alleviate tension in the lower back, which is especially beneficial for those who sit for prolonged periods. This exercise also promotes blood flow to the upper body, making it a great choice for a warm-up or cool-down routine.

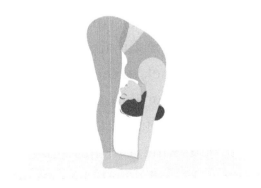

If you find yourself needing a visual reference for any of the exercises, a simple search on a video platform like YouTube, using the name of the pose, can offer you supplementary guidance. This way, you can ensure you're performing each movement correctly and safely.

Dynamic Leg Stretches

How to Perform Dynamic Leg Stretches

1. Starting Position: Stand upright with your feet hip-width apart. Keep your arms at your sides or place your hands on your hips for balance.

2. Forward Leg Swings: Begin with forward leg swings. Swing one leg forward and backward, gently increasing the range of motion. Keep your leg straight as you swing it, and avoid arching your back. Do this for about 30 seconds, then switch legs.

3. Side Leg Swings: Next, move to side leg swings. Stand sideways near a wall or a stable object for support. Swing your outside leg across the front of your body and then out to the side, again keeping the leg straight. Continue for about 30 seconds before switching to the other leg.

4. Lunging Stretch: Perform dynamic lunging stretches. Step forward into a lunge and lower your hips until your front thigh is parallel to the floor. Ensure your front knee doesn't go past your toes. Push back to the starting position and alternate legs. Continue for about 1 minute.

5. Rhythm and Breathing: Maintain a rhythmic pace and coordinate your breath with your movements. Inhale as you prepare for the stretch, and exhale as you execute the stretch.

Dynamic Leg Stretches

Tips
- Dynamic leg stretches should be performed in a controlled manner. Avoid jerky or overly forceful movements that could strain your muscles.
- Focus on warming up the muscles rather than stretching them to their limits. The goal is to prepare your muscles for more intense activity.
- As you progress, you can increase the speed and range of motion, but always listen to your body and stay within a comfortable range.
- Keep your core engaged during these stretches to support your back and improve balance.

Note
Dynamic leg stretches are ideal for warming up the leg muscles in motion, preparing them for a workout or physical activity. They help improve circulation, increase muscle temperature, and enhance flexibility, reducing the risk of injury during more strenuous exercises.

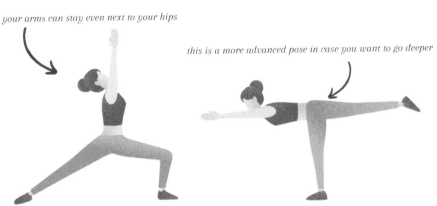

your arms can stay even next to your hips

this is a more advanced pose in case you want to go deeper

If you find yourself needing a visual reference for any of the exercises, a simple search on a video platform like YouTube, using the name of the pose, can offer you supplementary guidance. This way, you can ensure you're performing each movement correctly and safely.

Butterfly Stretch

How to Perform the Butterfly Stretch

1. Starting Position: Sit on the floor with your spine straight and tall. Bring the soles of your feet together in front of you, drawing your heels as close to your body as comfortable.
2. Knee Position: Allow your knees to fall out to the sides, feeling a stretch in your inner thighs. If your knees are high off the ground, that's okay – flexibility will improve over time.
3. Intensifying the Stretch: Gently press down on your thighs or knees with your elbows or hands for a deeper stretch, but be careful not to force them down.
4. Maintain the Position: Hold the stretch for 20-30 seconds, breathing deeply and steadily. Focus on relaxing your muscles with each exhale.
5. Avoid Bouncing: Keep the stretch static – avoid bouncing your knees up and down.
6. Exiting the Stretch: To release, slowly lift your knees, bring your legs together, and shake them out gently.

Butterfly Stretch

Tips

- Ensure that you're seated comfortably. You can sit on a cushion or folded blanket for added support.
- Keep your back straight throughout the stretch to prevent any strain on your spine.
- If you feel any pain or discomfort, ease off the stretch a bit. Stretching should involve a gentle pull, not pain.
- For an additional stretch, you can lean your torso forward from your hips while keeping your back straight. This motion deepens the stretch in your inner thighs and hips.
- As with any static stretch, focus on relaxing into the stretch rather than pushing too hard. Over time, your flexibility will naturally increase.

Note

The Butterfly Stretch is a fantastic static stretch for the inner thighs and hips. It's especially beneficial for those who require increased hip flexibility, such as runners, cyclists, or anyone who sits for long periods. Regular practice of this stretch can improve hip mobility, reduce tightness in the inner thighs, and promote overall lower body flexibility.

If you want a deeper stretch you can try this version

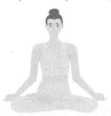

If you find yourself needing a visual reference for any of the exercises, a simple search on a video platform like YouTube, using the name of the pose, can offer you supplementary guidance. This way, you can ensure you're performing each movement correctly and safely.

Lunge with a Twist

How to Perform Lunge with a Twist

1. Starting Position: Stand with your feet together and your hands on your hips. Keep your back straight and your shoulders relaxed.
2. Step into a Lunge: Take a large step forward with your right foot, bending your knee to about a 90-degree angle. Your front thigh should be parallel to the floor, and your back leg should be straight with the heel lifted off the ground.
3. Perform the Twist: As you lunge, extend your arms out to the sides at shoulder height. Then, twist your upper body to the right, keeping your arms parallel to the floor. Turn your head to look over your right shoulder if it's comfortable.
4. Return to Starting Position: Untwist your upper body and bring your arms back to your sides. Push off your right foot to return to the starting position.
5. Repeat on the Other Side: Repeat the movement, this time stepping forward with your left foot and twisting to the left.
6. Rhythm and Breathing: Coordinate your movements with your breathing. Inhale as you step into the lunge and exhale as you twist.

Lunge with a Twist

Tips

- Keep your front knee aligned with your front ankle and ensure it doesn't extend past your toes to prevent strain.
- Engage your core muscles during the twist to support your spine and enhance the stretch.
- The twist should be gentle and controlled. Avoid over-rotating your torso.
- Keep your neck in a neutral position, in line with your spine, and avoid straining it as you turn your head.
- If balancing is challenging, perform the exercise near a wall or a chair for support.

Note

The Lunge with a Twist is an effective exercise for combining stretching and mobilization. It targets the leg muscles, hips, and spine, providing a dynamic stretch that enhances flexibility and encourages mobility in the torso. This exercise is particularly beneficial for loosening tight hip flexors and improving rotational movement in the upper body, making it a great addition to any warm-up or cool-down routine.

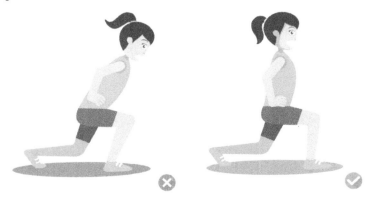

If you find yourself needing a visual reference for any of the exercises, a simple search on a video platform like YouTube, using the name of the pose, can offer you supplementary guidance. This way, you can ensure you're performing each movement correctly and safely.

BASIC EXERCISES

Pelvic Tilts

How to Perform Pelvic Tilts

1. Starting Position: Lie on your back on a flat surface (use a yoga mat for comfort). Bend your knees with your feet flat on the floor, hip-width apart. Keep your arms at your sides with palms facing down.

2. Neutral Spine: Start by establishing a neutral spine position. There should be a slight, natural curve in your lower back, and your spine should not be pressed into the floor.

3. Engage Your Core: Tighten your abdominal muscles, drawing your navel towards your spine. This engagement is crucial for the effectiveness of the exercise.

4. Tilt Your Pelvis: Exhale as you gently tilt your pelvis towards your ribcage. This movement will flatten your lower back against the floor. Avoid lifting your hips off the floor – the movement is small and controlled.

5. Return to Neutral: Inhale and slowly release the tilt, returning your pelvis to the neutral starting position.

6. Repetitions: Perform this movement for 10-15 repetitions, focusing on slow and controlled tilts.

Pelvic Tilts

Tips

- It's important to keep the rest of your body relaxed. The movement should be isolated to your pelvis and lower back.
- Keep your breath steady and synchronized with your movements – exhale during the tilt and inhale as you return to neutral.
- Don't rush the tilts. The effectiveness of pelvic tilts comes from the quality of the movement, not the quantity.
- As you get more comfortable with the exercise, you can hold the tilt for a few seconds before returning to the neutral position.

Note

Pelvic tilts are a fundamental exercise for strengthening the core and the lower back. They are particularly beneficial for improving lumbar spine stability, which can help alleviate lower back pain. This exercise is also a great starting point for building a stronger core, which is essential for overall body strength and injury prevention. Regular practice of pelvic tilts can lead to improved posture and a more supportive base for various physical activities.

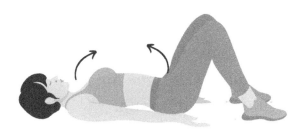

If you find yourself needing a visual reference for any of the exercises, a simple search on a video platform like YouTube, using the name of the pose, can offer you supplementary guidance. This way, you can ensure you're performing each movement correctly and safely.

Cat-Cow Stretch

How to Perform the Cat-Cow Stretch

1. Starting Position: Begin on your hands and knees in a tabletop position. Ensure your knees are set directly below your hips and your wrists, elbows, and shoulders are in line and perpendicular to the floor. Center your head in a neutral position, eyes looking at the floor.

2. Cow Pose: As you inhale, drop your belly towards the floor, lift your chin and chest, and gaze up toward the ceiling. In this position, you're making a concave shape with your spine.

3. Cat Pose: As you exhale, draw your belly to your spine and round your back toward the ceiling. The pose should look like a cat stretching its back. Release the crown of your head toward the floor, but don't force your chin to your chest.

4. Flowing Movement: Inhale, coming back into Cow Pose, and then exhale as you return to Cat Pose. Make the transition between these poses a smooth and fluid movement.

5. Rhythm and Breathing: Synchronize your movements with your breath, moving into Cow Pose on the inhale and into Cat Pose on the exhale. Continue for 1-2 minutes, following the natural rhythm of your breath.

Cat-Cow Stretch

Tips

- Keep your movements gentle and mindful. Do not rush the stretches or force your body into any positions that feel uncomfortable.
- Focus on the sensation of your spine arching and rounding. This exercise should feel good and help release tension in your back.
- Ensure that you keep your shoulders and knees in alignment to avoid any strain.
- If you have any neck issues, keep the head in line with the torso rather than dropping it back or forward.

Note

The Cat-Cow Stretch is excellent for enhancing spinal flexibility. It helps to gently stretch the spine, neck, and torso, while also massaging the organs in the belly. This exercise is a great way to start any workout routine as it warms up the body and brings increased awareness to the spine, a central area of movement in many exercises. Regular practice can lead to improved posture and relief from tension and stress in the back.

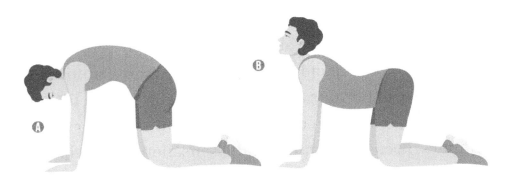

If you find yourself needing a visual reference for any of the exercises, a simple search on a video platform like YouTube, using the name of the pose, can offer you supplementary guidance. This way, you can ensure you're performing each movement correctly and safely.

Breath Awareness Exercise

How to Perform the Breath Awareness Exercise

1. Finding a Comfortable Position: Begin by finding a comfortable seated or lying down position. If seated, ensure your back is straight and your feet are flat on the floor. If lying down, lay flat on your back with your legs slightly apart and arms at your sides.

2. Relax Your Body: Close your eyes to help focus inward. Consciously relax your muscles, starting from your toes, moving up through your legs, torso, arms, and finally, your head.

3. Focus on Your Breathing: Place one hand on your chest and the other on your abdomen. This will help you focus on the movement of your diaphragm as you breathe.

4. Diaphragmatic Breathing: Inhale deeply through your nose, allowing your abdomen to rise as your lungs fill with air. Feel the hand on your abdomen rise, while the hand on your chest remains relatively still.

5. Exhale Slowly: Exhale slowly and completely through your mouth or nose, depending on what feels most comfortable. Feel the hand on your abdomen fall as you release the air.

6. Repeat: Continue to breathe deeply and slowly for several minutes. Focus your mind on the sensation of your breath entering and leaving your body, and the rise and fall of your abdomen.

Breath Awareness Exercise

Tips

- If your mind starts to wander, gently bring your focus back to your breathing. It's normal for the mind to drift, and the exercise includes returning your focus to your breath.
- Try to maintain a steady rhythm in your breathing, making your inhales and exhales of equal length.
- Diaphragmatic breathing not only aids in relaxation but also ensures efficient oxygen exchange and can improve respiratory and overall health.
- This exercise can be performed anytime you need to relax or refocus, such as before bed, upon waking up, or during breaks in your day.

Note

The Breath Awareness Exercise is centered on focusing on diaphragmatic breathing, which is a key component of stress reduction and relaxation. It encourages a deeper, more effective breathing pattern, which can have a calming effect on the nervous system. Regular practice can improve lung function, reduce stress levels, and enhance overall well-being. This exercise is also a foundational practice in many forms of meditation and yoga, emphasizing the connection between breath and mental clarity.

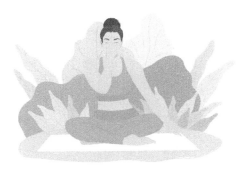

Balancing Table Pose

How to Perform the Balancing Table Pose

1. Starting Position: Begin on your hands and knees in a tabletop position. Position your wrists directly under your shoulders and your knees under your hips. Keep your back flat and your head and neck in a neutral position, looking down at the floor.

2. Extend Arm and Opposite Leg: Extend your right arm forward until it's in line with your torso while simultaneously stretching your left leg back until it's in line with your body. Keep both your extended arm and leg parallel to the floor.

3. Focus on Balance: Engage your core muscles to maintain balance. Try to keep your hips and shoulders squared to the floor.

4. Hold the Pose: Hold this position for a few seconds, focusing on stability and balance.

5. Return to Tabletop: Gently lower your extended arm and leg back to the tabletop position.

6. Repeat on the Opposite Side: Extend your left arm and right leg, following the same steps. Alternate sides for several repetitions.

Balancing Table Pose

Tips

- Keep your movements slow and controlled. Avoid any jerky movements, which can throw off your balance.
- If you find it difficult to balance, start by lifting just an arm or just a leg instead of both.
- Keep breathing steadily throughout the exercise. Holding your breath can make balancing more challenging.
- Focus your gaze on a fixed point on the floor to help maintain balance.

Note

Balancing Table Pose is excellent for improving balance and coordination. It strengthens the core, arms, and legs, and enhances focus and concentration. This pose is also beneficial for promoting better body awareness, as it requires you to be mindful of your alignment and movement. Regular practice of this pose can significantly improve your stability, which is beneficial for daily activities and other forms of exercise.

If you find yourself needing a visual reference for any of the exercises, a simple search on a video platform like YouTube, using the name of the pose, can offer you supplementary guidance. This way, you can ensure you're performing each movement correctly and safely.

Knee-to-Chest Stretch

How to Perform Knee-to-Chest Stretch

1. Starting Position: Lie on your back on a flat, comfortable surface. Extend your legs straight out and relax your upper body, with your arms resting at your sides.

2. Bringing Knee to Chest: Bend your right knee and gently pull it towards your chest using both hands. Clasp your hands either behind your thigh or on top of your shin (but not on the knee cap) for support.

3. Hold the Stretch: Once you've brought your knee as close to your chest as comfortably possible, hold the position. You should feel a gentle stretch in your lower back and hip. Maintain this hold for about 20-30 seconds.

4. Return to Starting Position: Gently release your right leg and extend it back to the floor. Take a moment to relax before switching to the other leg.

5. Repeat with the Other Leg: Perform the same stretch with your left knee, following the same steps.

6. Alternate Legs: Continue to alternate between your right and left legs for a few repetitions.

Knee-to-Chest Stretch

Tips

- Ensure that your movements are slow and controlled. Avoid any sudden pulling or jerking motions.
- Keep your lower back pressed against the floor throughout the stretch to protect it and maximize the stretch on your hips.
- Breathe deeply and steadily as you perform this stretch. Deep breathing helps relax your muscles and deepens the stretch.
- If you experience any pain or discomfort, especially in the back or knee, ease off the stretch a bit.

Note

The Knee-to-Chest Stretch is a simple yet effective exercise for relaxing the lower back and hips. It helps alleviate tension and stiffness in these areas, which is especially beneficial for individuals who sit for long periods or have lower back discomfort. This stretch can also aid in improving hip flexibility and promoting overall relaxation in the lower body. Regular practice can contribute to a greater range of motion and comfort in daily movements.

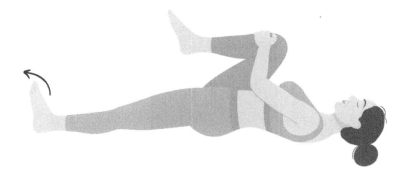

If you find yourself needing a visual reference for any of the exercises, a simple search on a video platform like YouTube, using the name of the pose, can offer you supplementary guidance. This way, you can ensure you're performing each movement correctly and safely.

INTERMEDIATE EXERCISES

Plank Pose

How to Perform Plank Pose

1. Starting Position: Begin in a tabletop position on your hands and knees. Place your wrists directly under your shoulders, and spread your fingers wide for a stable base.

2. Extend Your Legs: Step your feet back one at a time, extending your legs fully. Your body should form a straight line from your heels to the crown of your head.

3. Engage Your Core: Tighten your abdominal muscles to prevent your hips from sagging or lifting too high. Your body should be as straight as possible, resembling a plank.

4. Shoulder Position: Keep your shoulders engaged and away from your ears. Your neck should be in line with your spine, with your gaze down at the floor.

5. Hold the Pose: Maintain the plank position for 20-60 seconds, depending on your ability. Keep breathing steadily throughout the exercise.

6. To Release: To come out of the pose, either lower your knees to the floor or shift into a downward dog pose by lifting your hips up and back.

Plank Pose

Tips

- Ensure that your weight is evenly distributed between your hands and toes. Avoid putting too much pressure on your wrists.
- If holding a full plank is too challenging, modify by keeping your knees on the floor.
- Keep your legs active and your heels pressing back to maintain the integrity of the pose.
- To avoid straining your neck, keep your gaze fixed on a spot on the floor just in front of your hands.
- Practice regularly to gradually increase the duration of the pose.

Note

Plank Pose is a foundational exercise for building core and shoulder stability. It not only strengthens the abdominal muscles but also engages the shoulders, chest, legs, and back, making it an effective full-body exercise. Regular practice of Plank Pose can improve posture, enhance balance, and build endurance in the core muscles. This pose is also beneficial for supporting the spine and can be a key exercise for developing overall body strength and stability.

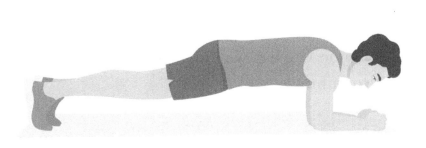

Bridge Pose

How to Perform Bridge Pose

1. Starting Position: Lie on your back on a comfortable, flat surface. Bend your knees and place your feet flat on the ground, hip-width apart. Extend your arms along the floor with your palms facing down, your fingertips should be lightly touching your heels.

2. Lifting the Hips: Press your feet and arms firmly into the ground as you lift your hips towards the ceiling. Keep your thighs and feet parallel – resist the urge to let your knees splay outward.

3. Engage Your Muscles: As you lift your hips, engage your glutes and hamstrings. Be mindful to not overarch your lower back. Instead, focus on creating a straight line from your shoulders to your knees.

4. Upper Body Position: Keep your neck relaxed and your gaze upwards. Do not turn your head side-to-side while in the pose.

5. Hold the Pose: Hold Bridge Pose for 30 seconds to 1 minute. Breathe deeply and maintain a steady lift through your hips.

6. Lowering Down: To release the pose, slowly lower your hips back to the floor. Once down, hug your knees to your chest for a gentle counter-stretch.

Bridge Pose

Tips

- Ensure that your movements are smooth and controlled. Avoid jerky movements, especially when lifting into and lowering from the pose.
- If you feel any strain in your neck or back, reduce the height of your lift or place a folded blanket under your shoulders for support.
- To increase the intensity, clasp your hands under your back and press your arms down, lifting your hips higher.
- Keep your breath steady throughout the pose. This will help maintain a balance between effort and relaxation.

Note

Bridge Pose, or Setu Bandhasana, is an effective exercise for strengthening the back, glutes, and hamstrings. It also helps open up the chest and shoulders, which can be beneficial for those who spend a lot of time sitting. This pose can aid in improving posture and alleviating lower back pain. Regular practice of Bridge Pose can enhance core stability and contribute to a stronger, more balanced lower body.

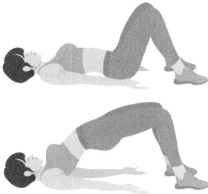

If you find yourself needing a visual reference for any of the exercises, a simple search on a video platform like YouTube, using the name of the pose, can offer you supplementary guidance. This way, you can ensure you're performing each movement correctly and safely.

Twisting Lunge

How to Perform Twisting Lunge

1. Starting Position: Stand with your feet together. Step your left foot back about three to four feet, keeping your left heel lifted off the floor. Align your right knee over your right ankle, so your right thigh is parallel to the floor in a lunge position.

2. Upper Body Position: Keep your torso upright and your core engaged. Extend your arms up overhead, keeping them in line with your ears.

3. Initiate the Twist: As you exhale, twist your upper body to the right. Bring your left elbow outside of your right knee. Press your palms together in a prayer position at your chest, and use your elbow against your knee to deepen the twist.

4. Gaze and Alignment: Keep your gaze forward or turn it up towards the ceiling if it's comfortable for your neck. Ensure that your hips remain square and facing forward – the twist should come from your torso, not your hips.

5. Hold the Pose: Hold the twisted lunge for about 20-30 seconds, breathing deeply. Stay strong and stable in your legs while twisting deeper with each exhale.

6. Return to Starting Position: Inhale as you unwind the twist, raising your arms back overhead. Step forward to return to the starting position.

7. Repeat on the Other Side: Repeat the same process on the other side, stepping back with your right foot and twisting to the left.

Twisting Lunge

Tips

- Ensure that your front knee doesn't extend past your toes to avoid strain.
- If balancing is challenging, perform the twist in a high lunge position without the elbow-to-knee connection.
- To modify, drop your back knee to the floor for a low lunge twist.
- Maintain a strong, active back leg throughout the pose for stability and support.
- Engage your abdominal muscles during the twist to enhance core strength and protect your spine.

Note

Twisting Lunge is an excellent exercise for enhancing core strength and flexibility. It combines the benefits of a lunge – strengthening the legs and stretching the hip flexors – with the advantages of a twist, which includes toning the abdominal muscles and improving spinal mobility. This pose also aids in digestion and detoxification, making it a beneficial addition to any intermediate-level workout routine. Regular practice can lead to a stronger, more flexible, and balanced body.

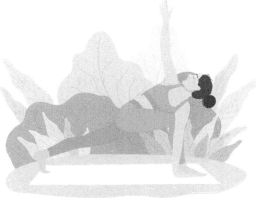

If you find yourself needing a visual reference for any of the exercises, a simple search on a video platform like YouTube, using the name of the pose, can offer you supplementary guidance. This way, you can ensure you're performing each movement correctly and safely.

Leg Raises

How to Perform Leg Raises

1. Starting Position: Lie flat on your back on a comfortable, firm surface. Keep your legs extended and together. Place your arms at your sides with palms facing down for stability, or you can place your hands under your lower back for additional support.

2. Engage Your Core: Tighten your abdominal muscles to stabilize your spine. Press your lower back into the floor to avoid arching.

3. Raise Your Legs: Slowly lift your legs off the ground, keeping them straight. Raise them to a 90-degree angle with your body, or as high as you can without bending your knees or arching your back.

4. Lower Your Legs: Slowly lower your legs back to the starting position. Control the movement to avoid any jerking or dropping.

5. Breathing: Exhale as you lift your legs and inhale as you lower them back down. Keep your breath steady and controlled.

6. Repetitions: Start with a set of 10-15 leg raises. As your strength improves, you can increase the number of repetitions or sets.

Leg Raises

Tips

- Focus on the quality of the movement rather than the quantity. It's more effective to do fewer controlled leg raises than many quick, uncontrolled ones.
- Keep your movements slow and controlled to maximize the engagement of your abdominal muscles.
- If you feel any strain in your lower back, reduce the range of motion, or bend your knees slightly.
- Avoid lifting your hips off the floor as you raise your legs. The movement should come solely from your hip flexors and abdominal muscles.

Note

Leg raises are an effective exercise for strengthening the abdominal and hip muscles. They specifically target the lower abdominals, a region often challenging to engage with other exercises. Leg raises also help in improving hip flexibility and can contribute to a stronger, more stable core. Regular practice can enhance core endurance, which is beneficial for posture, balance, and overall athletic performance.

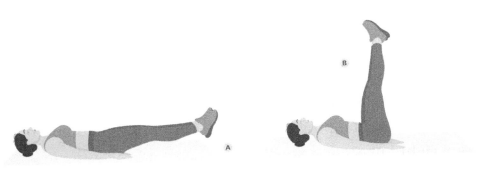

If you find yourself needing a visual reference for any of the exercises, a simple search on a video platform like YouTube, using the name of the pose, can offer you supplementary guidance. This way, you can ensure you're performing each movement correctly and safely.

Warrior II Pose

How to Perform Warrior II Pose

1. Starting Position: Begin standing with your feet together. Take a large step back with your right foot, keeping your left foot pointing forward. Your right foot should be turned outwards, approximately 90 degrees.

2. Aligning the Pose: Align your left heel with the arch of your right foot. Ensure your hips are open to the side, facing the same direction as your right foot.

3. Lowering into the Pose: Bend your left knee until it is directly over your left ankle, forming a right angle. Your right leg should remain straight.

4. Arm Position: Extend your arms out to the sides at shoulder height, keeping them parallel to the floor. Gaze over your left hand.

5. Holding the Pose: Hold this position, breathing deeply, for 30 seconds to 1 minute. Maintain a strong, grounded stance while keeping your upper body relaxed.

6. Return to Starting Position: To release the pose, straighten your left knee, lower your arms, and step your feet back together.

7. Repeat on the Other Side: Repeat the same process on the opposite side, stepping back with your left foot and bending your right knee.

Warrior II Pose

Tips

- Keep your front knee aligned with your front ankle to avoid straining the knee joint.
- Press down through the outer edge of your back foot for stability.
- Engage your core muscles to help maintain balance and support your upper body.
- Keep your shoulders relaxed and away from your ears, and your arms strong and active.
- If you feel unsteady, shorten your stance or perform the pose near a wall for support.

Note

Warrior II Pose, also known as Virabhadrasana II, is a powerful stance that builds lower body strength and balance. It targets the legs, hips, and ankles, while also stretching the chest and shoulders. This pose is excellent for improving stability and endurance, and it also encourages focus and concentration. Regular practice of Warrior II can enhance overall body alignment and posture.

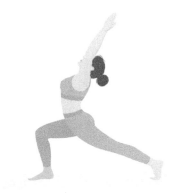 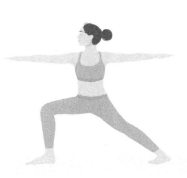

If you find yourself needing a visual reference for any of the exercises, a simple search on a video platform like YouTube, using the name of the pose, can offer you supplementary guidance. This way, you can ensure you're performing each movement correctly and safely.

ADVANCED EXERCISES

Handstand Practice

How to Perform Handstand Practice

1. Preparation: Begin by warming up your wrists, shoulders, and core muscles, as they will be extensively used in a handstand.

2. Starting Position: Start in a standing position near a wall for support. Bend forward and place your hands on the floor, shoulder-width apart, about a foot away from the wall.

3. Kick-Up: Step one foot closer to your hands, keeping the other leg extended. Gently kick up with the bent leg, followed by the extended leg, using the wall for support. Your goal is to get both legs up and your body in a straight vertical line.

4. Alignment: Keep your arms straight and engage your core muscles. Your body should be as straight as possible from your hands to your feet. Tuck your pelvis slightly to avoid arching your back.

5. Balancing: Once you're up, focus on finding your balance. Keep your gaze on the floor between your hands. Use your fingertips to make minor adjustments to your balance.

6. Hold the Pose: Try to hold the handstand for a few seconds to start, gradually increasing the duration as you gain strength and confidence.

7. To Exit: Gently lower your legs back to the floor, one at a time, returning to the standing position.

Handstand Practice

Tips

- It's essential to build up to a full handstand gradually. Begin with shorter attempts and use the wall for safety.
- Focus on keeping your body tight and aligned. This will help maintain balance and prevent injury.
- Breathing is important. Try to maintain steady and controlled breaths while in the handstand.
- Practice regularly. Consistency is key to building the strength and balance needed for a handstand.
- If you're new to handstands, consider practicing with a spotter or an experienced instructor.

Note

Handstand Practice is an advanced exercise that builds upper body strength and balance. It primarily targets the shoulders, arms, and core muscles. In addition to physical strength, handstands require and develop focus, body awareness, and confidence. Regular practice can significantly improve upper body conditioning, balance skills, and overall body control. As an inversion, it also provides the benefits of reversing the flow of gravity, which can be refreshing and energizing.

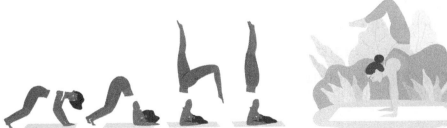

Advanced option

If you find yourself needing a visual reference for any of the exercises, a simple search on a video platform like YouTube, using the name of the pose, can offer you supplementary guidance. This way, you can ensure you're performing each movement correctly and safely.

Crow Pose

How to Perform Crow Pose

1. Starting Position: Begin in a squat position with your feet a few inches apart. If you have tight hips, your heels may lift off the ground – you can place a folded mat or blanket under them for support.

2. Hand Placement: Place your hands flat on the floor about shoulder-width apart, with fingers spread wide.

3. Knee and Arm Position: Press your knees into the back of your upper arms. Start to shift your weight forward, coming onto the balls of your feet.

4. Lift Off: Engage your core and lift your feet off the ground one at a time. Your gaze should be forward, not down. This will help with balance.

5. Balancing: Keep your elbows slightly bent. Balance your knees on your arms and your body weight on your hands. Try to bring your feet together behind you.

6. Hold the Pose: Hold Crow Pose for a few seconds to start, working up to longer as you gain strength and confidence. Keep breathing steadily.

7. To Release: Gently lower your feet back to the ground, returning to a squat position.

Crow Pose

Tips

- Crow Pose requires strength and balance, so don't be discouraged if it takes several attempts to get into the pose.
- Focus on engaging your core throughout the pose. This will help stabilize your body and make it easier to lift and hold your legs up.
- Keep your elbows in line with your wrists to maintain stability and prevent strain.
- Practice near a wall or cushion in front of you for safety, especially if you're worried about falling forward.
- Before attempting Crow Pose, warm up with wrist stretches and some core strengthening exercises.

Note

Crow Pose, or Bakasana, is an arm balancing pose that greatly enhances arm and core strength. It also improves focus, balance, and coordination. The pose strengthens the arms, wrists, and abdominal muscles, while also stretching the upper back and opening the groins. Regular practice of Crow Pose can develop mental and physical poise, as well as the confidence to attempt more challenging arm balances.

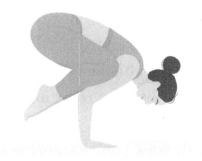

If you find yourself needing a visual reference for any of the exercises, a simple search on a video platform like YouTube, using the name of the pose, can offer you supplementary guidance. This way, you can ensure you're performing each movement correctly and safely.

Pigeon Pose

How to Perform Pigeon Pose

1. Starting Position: Begin in a tabletop position on your hands and knees.

2. Move into the Pose: Slide your right knee forward between your hands. Angle your right knee at two o'clock and place your right ankle near your left hip. Extend your left leg straight back behind you, keeping your hips square to the floor.

3. Adjust Your Position: If your right hip does not comfortably reach the floor, place a folded blanket or cushion underneath for support. This will help maintain alignment and prevent strain.

4. Upper Body Position: Initially, keep your torso upright and hands placed on the floor for balance. Inhale deeply as you lengthen your spine.

5. Forward Bend (Optional): For a deeper stretch, exhale and slowly walk your hands forward, bringing your torso down towards the floor. Rest your forehead on your hands or the floor, whichever is comfortable.

6. Hold the Pose: Stay in this position for 30 seconds to a minute, allowing your body to relax and sink deeper into the stretch with each exhale.

7. To Release: Gently walk your hands back, lifting your torso. Slide your right knee back to return to a tabletop position. Repeat the pose with your left knee forward.

Pigeon Pose

Tips

- Ensure that your back leg is aligned straight behind you and not angled to one side.
- Keep your front foot flexed to protect your knee joint.
- Breathing is key in Pigeon Pose. Deep, steady breaths will help you relax into the stretch.
- If you feel any sharp pain, especially in the knee, come out of the pose and consider a modified version or a different hip-opening exercise.
- Regularly practicing Pigeon Pose on both sides can help maintain balance in your hip flexibility.

Note

Pigeon Pose, or Eka Pada Rajakapotasana, is a deep stretching pose for the hips and glutes. It is highly beneficial for people who spend long periods sitting, as it effectively opens the hip flexors and rotators. The pose also stretches the thighs, groin, and psoas, and can relieve tension and tightness in the lower back. Regular practice of Pigeon Pose can enhance flexibility in the lower body, promote circulation, and contribute to overall hip health.

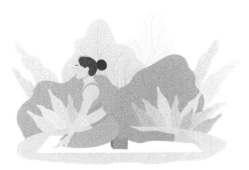

If you find yourself needing a visual reference for any of the exercises, a simple search on a video platform like YouTube, using the name of the pose, can offer you supplementary guidance. This way, you can ensure you're performing each movement correctly and safely.

Boat Pose

How to Perform Boat Pose

1. Starting Position: Sit on the floor with your knees bent and your feet flat on the ground. Lean back slightly, but keep your spine straight.

2. Lift Your Feet: Engage your core muscles and lift your feet off the floor, bringing your shins parallel to the floor. This is the half-boat pose, a good starting point for beginners.

3. Extend Your Arms: Stretch your arms forward, parallel to the floor with palms facing each other. Keep your shoulders relaxed and away from your ears.

4. Full Boat Pose (Optional): If you feel stable, straighten your legs, bringing your body into a 'V' shape. Keep your chest open and your spine straight.

5. Hold the Pose: Whether in half-boat or full boat pose, try to hold the position for 10-30 seconds, depending on your ability. Breathe steadily.

6. To Release: Exhale as you lower your legs and return to the starting position.

Boat Pose

Tips

- Focus on maintaining a straight back throughout the pose. Avoid rounding your spine.
- If you find it challenging to balance, keep your hands on the floor beside your hips for support.
- Engage your abdominal muscles to support your spine and help maintain balance.
- If you experience any discomfort in your lower back, try bending your knees or reducing the angle between your torso and legs.
- Over time, as your core strength improves, try to increase the duration of the pose or progress to the full boat pose.

Note

Boat Pose, or Navasana, is an excellent exercise for challenging and strengthening the core muscles, including the abdominals, hip flexors, and lower back. It also helps improve balance and stability. Regular practice of Boat Pose can enhance overall core strength, which is crucial for good posture and stability in various physical activities and exercises. Additionally, it can stimulate the kidneys, thyroid, prostate glands, and intestines, helping with digestion.

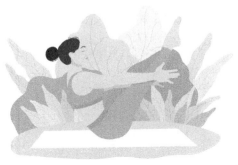

If you find yourself needing a visual reference for any of the exercises, a simple search on a video platform like YouTube, using the name of the pose, can offer you supplementary guidance. This way, you can ensure you're performing each movement correctly and safely.

Inverted Shoulder Stand

How to Perform Inverted Shoulder Stand

1. Starting Position: Begin by lying on your back on a comfortable surface. Place your arms at your sides, palms down for support.

2. Lift Your Legs: Bend your knees and bring them towards your chest. Gradually lift your hips off the floor, using your hands to support your lower back.

3. Straighten Your Body: Extend your legs upward, straightening your spine so that your body forms a straight line. Your weight should be supported by your shoulders, arms, and neck, not your head or neck.

4. Alignment: Keep your legs and spine as vertical as possible. Your chin should be tucked into your chest.

5. Hold the Pose: Maintain the pose for 30 seconds to a few minutes, depending on your comfort and experience level. Breathe deeply and steadily.

6. To Release: Gently lower your legs over your head into a plow pose, if possible, then slowly roll your spine back onto the floor, one vertebra at a time, using your hands for support.

Inverted Shoulder Stand

Tips

- Start with shorter durations and gradually increase as you become more comfortable with the pose.
- Keep the neck and head still throughout the pose to avoid strain. All the movement should come from the spine and hips.
- If you are a beginner, consider practicing near a wall or with the assistance of an experienced instructor.
- Avoid this pose if you have high blood pressure, neck issues, or are currently experiencing headaches or heart problems.

Note

Inverted Shoulder Stand, or Sarvangasana, is a powerful inversion known for its numerous benefits. It is particularly effective in improving circulation and balance. The pose encourages blood flow from the legs and pelvis back to the heart and then circulates it throughout the lungs and upper body, which can be revitalizing. Additionally, it strengthens the shoulders, back, and core muscles, enhancing overall stability and posture. Regular practice of Inverted Shoulder Stand can also help in calming the mind and relieving stress.

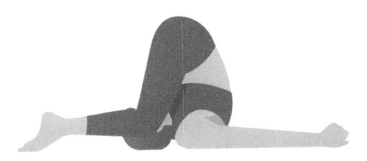

If you find yourself needing a visual reference for any of the exercises, a simple search on a video platform like YouTube, using the name of the pose, can offer you supplementary guidance. This way, you can ensure you're performing each movement correctly and safely.

3

DAILY ROUTINES

Welcome to the Daily Routines section of "Somatic Exercises for Weight Loss." This part of the book is designed to provide you with a structured approach to incorporating the exercises you've learned into your daily life. Each of the 30 routines has been carefully crafted to ensure a balanced workout, catering to different fitness levels and focusing on various aspects of physical well-being. The routines combine warm-up exercises, dynamic and static stretching, basic movements, intermediate challenges, and advanced poses to create a holistic workout experience. Whether you're looking to enhance your core strength, improve your flexibility, build balance and coordination, or engage in a relaxing and rejuvenating exercise session, these routines offer something for everyone.

How to Use These Routines:

 - Flexibility in Practice: Feel free to adapt these routines to suit your schedule and fitness level. You can shorten or lengthen the duration of each exercise or the entire routine as needed.

 - Progression and Variation: As you become more comfortable with the exercises, challenge yourself by increasing repetitions, extending hold times, or incorporating more advanced versions of the exercises.

- Listen to Your Body: Always be mindful of how your body feels during each exercise. If something doesn't feel right, make adjustments or skip the exercise. Safety and comfort are paramount.

- Consistency is Key: Try to incorporate these exercises into your daily routine. Even a few minutes each day can make a significant difference in your overall health and well-being.

- Track Your Progress: Consider keeping an exercise diary to note down which routines you've done, how you felt before and after, and any progress you observe over time.

- Enjoy the Routines: If a particular exercise feels too challenging, it's perfectly okay to replace it with one you were comfortable with from a previous day. Additionally, once you've completed all 30 days, you can revisit and repeat the routines in any order that suits your preference and comfort level. This flexibility ensures your exercise regimen stays enjoyable, adaptable, and aligned with your ongoing wellness journey.

Each routine is a stepping stone towards better health and fitness. As you embark on this journey, remember that the goal is not only to improve your physical fitness but also to enhance your mind-body connection, nurture your mental well-being, and enjoy the process of self-care.

Let's get started on this path to a healthier, more balanced you!

Your 30 Daily Routines

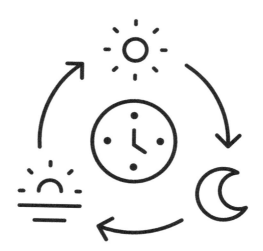

Embrace each day as a new opportunity to strengthen your body and mind.

Day 1: Core Activation and Balance

Warm-Up	**Jogging on the Spot (5 mins)**
Basic	**Cat-Cow Stretch (2 mins)**
Intermediate	**Plank Pose (1 min)**
Advanced	**Boat Pose (30 secs)**
Cool-Down	**Breath Awareness Exercise (5 mins)**

Your journey to wellness begins with a single step.

Day 2: Lower Body Strength

Warm-Up	Hip Circles (5 mins)
Basic	Pelvic Tilts (2 mins)
Intermediate	Warrior II Pose (1 min each side)
Advanced	Pigeon Pose (2 mins each side)
Cool-Down	Butterfly Stretch (5 mins)

Believe in the power of your own strength.

Day 3: Upper Body and Core Focus

Warm-Up	Arm Swings (5 mins)
Basic	Knee-to-Chest Stretch (2 mins)
Intermediate	Twisting Lunge (1 min each side)
Advanced	Crow Pose (30 secs)
Cool-Down	Spinal Twists (5 mins)

Every moment of movement is a step towards a better you.

Day 4: Full Body Conditioning

Warm-Up	**Dynamic Leg Stretches (5 mins)**
Basic	**Balancing Table Pose (2 mins)**
Intermediate	**Bridge Pose (1 min)**
Advanced	**Inverted Shoulder Stand (1 min)**
Cool-Down	**Standing Toe Touches (5 mins)**

Balance in the body brings harmony to the soul.

Day 5 : Flexibility and Core

Warm-Up	Arm and Shoulder Stretch (5 mins)
Basic	Cat-Cow Stretch (2 mins)
Intermediate	Leg Raises (2 mins)
Advanced	Handstand Practice (as long as comfortable)
Cool-Down	Butterfly Stretch (5 mins)

Transform challenges into opportunities for growth.

Day 6: Hip Mobility and Strength

Warm-Up	Hip Circles (5 mins)
Basic	Pelvic Tilts (2 mins)
Intermediate	Plank Pose (1 min)
Advanced	Pigeon Pose (2 mins each side)
Cool-Down	Knee-to-Chest Stretch (5 mins)

Find strength in stillness and calm in action.

Day 7: Core and Balance Challenge

Warm-Up	Jogging on the Spot (5 mins)
Basic	Breath Awareness Exercise (5 mins)
Intermediate	Twisting Lunge (1 min each side)
Advanced	Boat Pose (30 secs)
Cool-Down	Spinal Twists (5 mins)

Your potential is limitless when you listen to your body.

Day 8: Lower Body Focus

Warm-Up	**Dynamic Leg Stretches (5 mins)**
Basic	**Knee-to-Chest Stretch (2 mins)**
Intermediate	**Warrior II Pose (1 min each side)**
Advanced	**Inverted Shoulder Stand (1 min)**
Cool-Down	**Cat-Cow Stretch (5 mins)**

Flexibility in the body mirrors flexibility in life.

Day 9: Upper Body and Core

Warm-Up	Arm Swings (5 mins)
Basic	Balancing Table Pose (2 mins)
Intermediate	Bridge Pose (1 min)
Advanced	Crow Pose (30 secs)
Cool-Down	Butterfly Stretch (5 mins)

Today's efforts are tomorrow's rewards.

Day 10: Flexibility and Strength

Warm-Up	Standing Toe Touches (5 mins)
Basic	Cat-Cow Stretch (2 mins)
Intermediate	Plank Pose (1 min)
Advanced	Handstand Practice (as long as comfortable)
Cool-Down	Breath Awareness Exercise (5 mins)

Let your breath be your guide to inner peace.

Day 11: Core and Hip Mobility

Warm-Up	Hip Circles (5 mins)
Basic	Pelvic Tilts (2 mins)
Intermediate	Leg Raises (2 mins)
Advanced	Pigeon Pose (2 mins each side)
Cool-Down	Spinal Twists (5 mins)

Physical strength paves the way for mental resilience.

Day 12: Core and Balance Challenge

Warm-Up	Jogging on the Spot (5 mins)
Basic	Breath Awareness Exercise (5 mins)
Intermediate	Twisting Lunge (1 min each side)
Advanced	Boat Pose (30 secs)
Cool-Down	Spinal Twists (5 mins)

Embrace the journey of self-discovery through movement.

Day 13: Lower Body Focus

Warm-Up	**Dynamic Leg Stretches (5 mins)**
Basic	**Knee-to-Chest Stretch (2 mins)**
Intermediate	**Warrior II Pose (1 min each side)**
Advanced	**Inverted Shoulder Stand (1 min)**
Cool-Down	**Cat-Cow Stretch (5 mins)**

In every stretch, find a space for personal growth.

Day 14: Upper Body and Core

Warm-Up	**Arm Swings (5 mins)**
Basic	**Balancing Table Pose (2 mins)**
Intermediate	**Bridge Pose (1 min)**
Advanced	**Crow Pose (30 secs)**
Cool-Down	**Butterfly Stretch (5 mins)**

Each day is a chance to create a healthier you.

Day 15 : Core Activation and Balance

Warm-Up	Jogging on the Spot (5 mins)
Basic	Cat-Cow Stretch (2 mins)
Intermediate	Plank Pose (1 min)
Advanced	Boat Pose (30 secs)
Cool-Down	Breath Awareness Exercise (5 mins)

Let mindfulness be your foundation for change.

Day 16: Lower Body Strength

Warm-Up	Hip Circles (5 mins)
Basic	Pelvic Tilts (2 mins)
Intermediate	Warrior II Pose (1 min each side)
Advanced	Pigeon Pose (2 mins each side)
Cool-Down	Butterfly Stretch (5 mins)

Your body is a temple: honor it with movement and care.

Day 17: Upper Body and Core Focus

Warm-Up	Arm Swings (5 mins)
Basic	Knee-to-Chest Stretch (2 mins)
Intermediate	Twisting Lunge (1 min each side)
Advanced	Crow Pose (30 secs)
Cool-Down	Spinal Twists (5 mins)

In the balance of body and mind, find your true center.

Day 18: Hip Mobility and Strength

Warm-Up	Hip Circles (5 mins)
Basic	Pelvic Tilts (2 mins)
Intermediate	Plank Pose (1 min)
Advanced	Pigeon Pose (2 mins each side)
Cool-Down	Knee-to-Chest Stretch (5 mins)

Transform your challenges into victories, one pose at a time.

Day 19: Core and Balance Challenge

Warm-Up	Jogging on the Spot (5 mins)
Basic	Breath Awareness Exercise (5 mins)
Intermediate	Twisting Lunge (1 min each side)
Advanced	Boat Pose (30 secs)
Cool-Down	Spinal Twists (5 mins)

Empower yourself through the discipline of practice.

Day 20: Lower Body Focus

Warm-Up	**Dynamic Leg Stretches (5 mins)**
Basic	**Knee-to-Chest Stretch (2 mins)**
Intermediate	**Warrior II Pose (1 min each side)**
Advanced	**Inverted Shoulder Stand (1 min)**
Cool-Down	**Cat-Cow Stretch (5 mins)**

Every exercise is a love letter to your body.

Day 21: Core Activation and Balance

Warm-Up	Jogging on the Spot (5 mins)
Basic	Cat-Cow Stretch (2 mins)
Intermediate	Plank Pose (1 min)
Advanced	Boat Pose (30 secs)
Cool-Down	Breath Awareness Exercise (5 mins)

Find joy in the journey, not just the destination.

Day 22: Lower Body Strength

Warm-Up	Hip Circles (5 mins)
Basic	Pelvic Tilts (2 mins)
Intermediate	Warrior II Pose (1 min each side)
Advanced	Pigeon Pose (2 mins each side)
Cool-Down	Butterfly Stretch (5 mins)

Strength isn't just physical: it's a state of mind.

Day 23: Hip Mobility and Strength

Warm-Up	Hip Circles (5 mins)
Basic	Pelvic Tilts (2 mins)
Intermediate	Plank Pose (1 min)
Advanced	Pigeon Pose (2 mins each side)
Cool-Down	Knee-to-Chest Stretch (5 mins)

Let your fitness journey be a reflection of self-love.

Day 24: Core and Balance Challenge

Warm-Up	Jogging on the Spot (5 mins)
Basic	Breath Awareness Exercise (5 mins)
Intermediate	Twisting Lunge (1 min each side)
Advanced	Boat Pose (30 secs)
Cool-Down	Spinal Twists (5 mins)

In harmony with your body, find peace for your mind.

Day 25: Lower Body Focus

Warm-Up	**Dynamic Leg Stretches (5 mins)**
Basic	**Knee-to-Chest Stretch (2 mins)**
Intermediate	**Warrior II Pose (1 min each side)**
Advanced	**Inverted Shoulder Stand (1 min)**
Cool-Down	**Cat-Cow Stretch (5 mins)**

Challenge yourself to reach new heights of well-being.

Day 26: Upper Body and Core

Warm-Up	**Arm Swings (5 mins)**
Basic	**Balancing Table Pose (2 mins)**
Intermediate	**Bridge Pose (1 min)**
Advanced	**Crow Pose (30 secs)**
Cool-Down	**Butterfly Stretch (5 mins)**

Your journey to wellness is a path of self-love and discovery.

Day 27: Flexibility and Strength

Warm-Up	Standing Toe Touches (5 mins)
Basic	Cat-Cow Stretch (2 mins)
Intermediate	Plank Pose (1 min)
Advanced	Handstand Practice (as long as comfortable)
Cool-Down	Breath Awareness Exercise (5 mins)

Mindfulness in motion creates harmony within.

Day 28: Core and Hip Mobility

Warm-Up	Hip Circles (5 mins)
Basic	Pelvic Tilts (2 mins)
Intermediate	Leg Raises (2 mins)
Advanced	Pigeon Pose (2 mins each side)
Cool-Down	Spinal Twists (5 mins)

Your greatest strength lies in the commitment to your health.

Day 29: Upper Body and Core

Warm-Up	Arm Swings (5 mins)
Basic	Cat-Cow Stretch (2 mins)
Intermediate	Bridge Pose (1 min)
Advanced	Crow Pose (30 secs)
Cool-Down	Butterfly Stretch (5 mins)

Embrace the transformative power of consistent practice.

Day 30: Flexibility and Strength

Warm-Up	**Standing Toe Touches (5 mins)**
Basic	**Pelvic Tilts (2 mins)**
Intermediate	**Plank Pose (1 min)**
Advanced	**Handstand Practice (as long as comfortable)**
Cool-Down	**Breath Awareness Exercise (5 mins)**

4

NUTRITIONAL ADVICE FOR SUPPORTING WEIGHT LOSS

Adopting a healthy approach to eating is a crucial component of any weight loss journey. While exercise plays a significant role in shaping your body and improving overall health, nutrition is equally important. The following guide offers essential nutritional advice aimed at supporting weight loss. However, remember that each individual's dietary needs are unique. It's highly recommended to consult a registered dietitian or nutritionist for personalized advice.

Understanding Calories

- Caloric Deficit for Weight Loss: Weight loss essentially occurs when you consume fewer calories than your body burns. Creating a caloric deficit, either by eating less, exercising more, or both, is vital.
- Quality Over Quantity: Focus on nutrient-dense foods rather than just counting calories. Foods rich in vitamins, minerals, and fiber will nourish your body and keep you fuller for longer.

Macronutrients Balance

- Proteins: Include lean proteins like chicken, fish, legumes, and tofu in your diet. Proteins are essential for muscle repair, especially after workouts, and can keep you feeling full.

- Carbohydrates: Opt for complex carbs like whole grains, fruits, and vegetables. They provide energy and are packed with nutrients and fiber, aiding digestion and providing sustained energy.

- Fats: Don't shy away from healthy fats found in avocados, nuts, seeds, and olive oil. They're vital for brain health and help in nutrient absorption.

Hydration

- Water is Key: Drinking adequate water is essential for weight loss. It boosts metabolism, helps in digestion, and can reduce the feeling of hunger.

- Limit Sugary Drinks: Reduce intake of sugary drinks, including sodas and store-bought juices. They add empty calories and can disrupt your weight loss efforts.

Meal Planning and Portion Control

- Regular, Balanced Meals: Eat at regular intervals to keep your metabolism steady. Skipping meals can lead to overeating later.

- Portion Sizes: Be mindful of portion sizes. Eating directly from large packages can lead to unintentional overeating.

Fruits and Vegetables

- Daily Intake: Aim to fill half your plate with fruits and vegetables. They are low in calories but high in fiber, vitamins, and minerals.

- Variety: Eat a wide variety of fruits and vegetables. Different colors provide different nutrients.

OLIVIA WELLNESS

Limiting Unhealthy Foods
- Reduced Processed Foods: Minimize consumption of processed foods, which are often high in calories, sugar, and unhealthy fats.
- Smart Snacking: Choose healthy snacks like fruits, nuts, or yogurt. Avoid snacking out of boredom or stress.

Mindful Eating
- Listen to Your Body: Eat when you're hungry and stop when you're full. Learn to differentiate between actual hunger and emotional eating.
- Enjoy Your Meals: Eat slowly and without distraction. It takes time for your brain to register fullness.

Consistency and Sustainability
- Long-Term Lifestyle Changes: Focus on making sustainable changes to your diet rather than temporary diets.
- Forgive Slip-Ups: Everyone has moments of indulgence. The key is to get back on track without guilt.

Seeking Professional Advice
- Consult a Professional: For a diet tailored to your individual needs, lifestyle, and health conditions, consult a dietitian or a nutritionist. They can provide valuable insights and structured meal plans.
- Medical Conditions: If you have any medical conditions or are on medication, it's crucial to seek professional advice before making significant dietary changes.

Nutrition plays a vital role in weight loss and overall well-being. By making mindful choices about what and how much to eat and ensuring a balanced intake of all nutrients, you can support your weight loss journey effectively. Remember, the goal is not just to lose weight but to nourish and respect your body. Adopting a balanced approach to nutrition is vital to long-term success and health.

AFTERWORD

As we draw to a close on "Somatic Exercises for Weight Loss," let's take a moment to reflect on the path we've journeyed together. This book has been more than a guide to shedding pounds; it's been a holistic exploration of wellness, intertwining the physical, mental, and nutritional aspects of health. From the outset, we delved into the world of somatic exercises, a realm where mindful movement and bodily awareness converge. These exercises aren't just about physical agility or strength; they're about developing a deeper understanding and connection with your body. By practicing movements like the gentle Cat-Cow Stretch, the stabilizing Warrior II Pose, or the core-engaging Boat Pose, you've embarked on a journey of not just physical fitness but also mental and emotional well-being. But our journey didn't stop at physical exercises. We explored the vast and crucial world of nutrition, underscoring that what we consume is as integral to our health as how we move. This wasn't about strict dieting or arbitrary food choices; it was about understanding your body's nutritional needs, the importance of balanced meals, and the profound impact that our eating habits have on our overall health. By integrating these dietary guidelines into your everyday life, you've started nourishing your body with the respect and care it deserves.

Afterword

Throughout this book, the themes of persistence and adaptability have been recurring. The journey to wellness is rarely straightforward; it's a path marked with both challenges and triumphs. The routines and advice provided offer a framework, yet they are imbued with the flexibility to adapt to your changing needs and circumstances. In this journey, every small step counts, and every bit of progress is worth celebrating. Now, as you continue on your path to wellness, remember that this is a journey of self-discovery and improvement. Your relationship with your body is deeply personal, and nurturing this connection requires patience, dedication, and compassion. The road to wellness is ongoing, and along the way, you'll learn more about yourself, your strengths, and areas where you can grow. In the spirit of this journey, I encourage you to maintain the practices and principles you've learned here. Keep exploring the depths of somatic exercises, listen to your body's needs, feed it thoughtfully, and most importantly, approach your wellness journey with kindness and an open heart. Remember, the ultimate goal is not just weight loss but achieving a state of holistic health and harmony within yourself. As you move forward, carry with you the lessons and experiences from this book. Let them be your guide and companion in your continuous quest for a healthier, more balanced, and fulfilling life. The path to wellness is uniquely yours, and every step you take on this path is a celebration of your commitment to your well-being. In closing, I would like to extend my heartfelt thanks to you for dedicating your time and energy to reading "Somatic Exercises for Weight Loss." Your commitment to enhancing your health and well-being is commendable, and I hope that this book has provided you with valuable insights and tools to support you on your wellness journey.

If you found this book helpful, please consider leaving a review on Amazon. Your feedback is not only greatly appreciated, but it also helps others discover this resource and embark on their paths to health and wellness. Sharing your experience and the impact this book has had on your journey can be incredibly inspiring and motivating to others looking to make similar changes in their lives.

Thank you once again for choosing this book as a companion on your wellness journey. Here's to your continued health and happiness!

APPENDIX

Glossary of Terms

1. Somatic Exercises: Physical movements focused on internal sensation and awareness, aimed at improving mind-body connection and holistic wellness.

2. Caloric Deficit: A state where you consume fewer calories than your body expends, leading to weight loss.

3. Macronutrients: The three main types of nutrients used by the body for energy, namely carbohydrates, proteins, and fats.

4. Diaphragmatic Breathing: A deep breathing technique that involves fully engaging the stomach, abdominal muscles, and diaphragm.

5. Mindful Eating: The practice of being fully attentive to the food and drink you consume, being aware of the taste, texture, and effects on the body.

6. Core Muscles: The muscles located in the abdomen, lower back, hips, and pelvis, which are essential for stability and balance.

7. Flexibility: The ability of muscles and joints to move through their full range of motion.

8. Balance: The ability to maintain the body's center of mass over its base of support.

9. Proprioception: The sense of self-movement and body position, often referred to as the "sixth sense."

Additional Resources and References

1. Books:

- "Yoga Anatomy" by Leslie Kaminoff and Amy Matthews – A comprehensive guide to yoga poses and their effects on the body.

- "The Complete Guide to Yin Yoga" by Bernie Clark – Detailed exploration of Yin Yoga for those looking to deepen their practice.

2. Websites:

- Yoga Journal (yogajournal.com) – Offers extensive resources on yoga, including detailed pose instructions and health benefits.

- Nutrition.gov (nutrition.gov) – A reliable source for nutritional advice, dietary guidelines, and healthy eating resources.

3. Apps:

- MyFitnessPal – A helpful tool for tracking diet and exercise, helping you understand and manage your caloric intake.

- Headspace – Offers guided meditation sessions, including exercises focused on mindful eating and stress reduction.

4. Professional Organizations:

- American Council on Exercise (acefitness.org) – Provides information on fitness education, certifications, and health and wellness tips.

- Academy of Nutrition and Dietetics (eatright.org) – The largest organization of food and nutrition professionals, offering nutritional advice and resources.

By exploring these additional resources, you can further enrich your understanding and practice of somatic exercises, nutrition, and overall wellness. Each resource offers unique insights and tools to support you in your journey to a healthier lifestyle. Remember, the path to wellness is a continuous journey of learning and growth.

Thank you Again.

Made in United States
North Haven, CT
16 January 2024

47539817R00075